Lose Weight Without The Wait

How To Lose Weight and Create A Body You Love Without Exercise

By
Jane Mukami

Lose Weight Without The Wait

© 2023 Jane Mukami

All rights reserved.

No part of this publication may be reproduced, distributed or transmitted in any form or by any means, including photocopying, recording, or other electronic or mechanical methods, without the prior written permission of the publisher, except in the case of brief quotations embodied in critical reviews and certain other noncommercial uses permitted by copyright law.

Although the author and publisher have made every effort to ensure that the information in this book was correct at press time, the author and publisher do not assume and hereby disclaim any liability to any party for any loss, damage, or disruption caused by errors or omissions, whether such errors or omissions result from negligence, accident, or any other cause.

Adherence to all applicable laws and regulations, including international, federal, state, and local governing professional licensing, business practices, advertising, and all other aspects of doing business in the US, Canada, or any other jurisdiction, is the sole responsibility of the reader and consumer.

Neither the author nor the publisher assumes any responsibility or liability whatsoever on behalf of the consumer or reader of this material. Any per-ceived slight of any individual or organization is purely unintentional.

The resources in this book are provided for informational purposes only. They should not be used to replace the specialized training and professional judgment of a health care or mental health care professional.

Neither the author nor the publisher can be held responsible for using the information provided within this book. Please always consult a trained professional before deciding to treat yourself or others.

For more information, e-mail jane@janemukami.com

ISBN:979-8-9888883-8-3 (Paperback)

Get Your Free Gift!

Thanks for getting this book. As a token of my appreciation, claim your free copy of the *Flat Belly Blueprint: How To Stubborn Lose Belly Fat*.

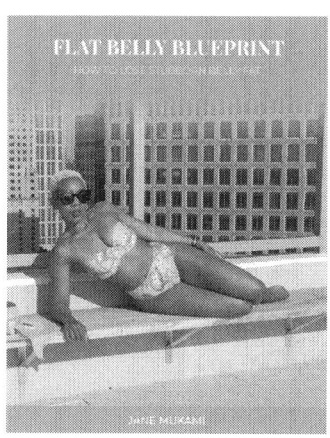

You can get a copy by scanning
the QR code below or visiting the link.

https://www.loseweightwithoutthewait.com/free-gift

DEDICATION

To all the women struggling to lose weight and can't seem to find the motivation or a successful way forward, this book is dedicated to you. Through its pages, embark on a journey towards greater self-esteem that won't involve struggling to lose weight. Be kind to yourself as you walk through this empowering experience. This book is your companion to losing weight so you can learn to love yourself and discover an improved version of you!

Table of Contents

Dedication vii

Introduction xi

Chapter 1: HELP! I'm Overweight 1

Chapter 2: What's Eating You? What's Happening Now? 13

Chapter 3: Your Diet Failed…Again 25

Chapter 4: Don't Do That, Do This! 35

Chapter 5: Fuel For The Fire 45

Chapter 6: First-class Body 55

Chapter 7: Body Upgrade 65

Chapter 8: Structured Eating 77

Chapter 9: The Best Hack Ever 89

Chapter 10: Weight Loss Method Final Notes 97

Bonus Chapter: Why You Shouldn't Give Up 105

Author's Bio 117

References 119

INTRODUCTION

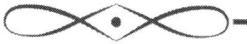

Can you imagine, loving the body "you see" when you look in the mirror and the body "they see" from the unedited pictures on your social media timeline? What if I told you that you no longer have to make excuses to skip social gatherings in fear of how you look to others? How wonderful would it be to put your clothes on with ease and without girdles or shapewear?

In this book, I will teach you how to lose weight with ease and keep the weight off so you can love your body, feel confident being around others, and enjoy a happy social life without feeling self-conscious.

I am Jane Mukami, a four-time award-winning nutrition-based weight loss coach and a graduate of the Harvard School of Medicine's Executive Program in Health & Wellness. I help women who feel trapped in bodies they don't like to increase confidence and look good naked by losing weight and learning how to keep it off. I believe that not only do we increase our life span by achieving our weight loss goals, but we also look and feel good about our bodies and show up as the best versions of ourselves to maximize our potential.

My Weight Loss Journey

I was exhausted, with dark circles under my eyes. My belly was pudgy and flowed onto my thighs; my sides started to fold over, like Bibendum the Michelin man's; my breasts spilled over my tight bra as if imprisoned and fighting to break free. It was a struggle; the bra was losing. I was trying to fit into a pair of pants that had been too big just six weeks prior, and they ripped! Ripped! Can you believe it?

Confusion, overwhelm, doubt, fear, and anger struck all at once. *"Who is this?"* I asked myself, *"How did I get here?"*

My recent divorce had taken its toll on me and left me feeling like a failure in all of life's departments. I became an emotional eater, gorging on food to suppress my pain and negative emotions.

Standing in front of the mirror that morning in April 2008, a ripped pair of pants was my much-needed wake-up call. I knew I had to lose weight, fall back in love with myself, and commit to taking control of my life once again.

Determination and Fad Diets

After ripping my pants earlier that morning, I decided to take matters into my own hands. First, I started going to the gym, hired a personal trainer, and enrolled in a boot camp. Without results, I hired another trainer, P90x, Slim-in-6, kickboxing, started outdoor running, and participated in half-marathons. Yet, my weight didn't budge.

I hired a third trainer, tried the grapefruit, tomato and starvation diet, started juicing, and added hydro-colon therapy. Before I knew it, two years had passed, and I had only lost four pounds. I felt at my lowest. Liposuction was my next solution since nothing else had worked. I met with a surgeon, paid a deposit, and began preparing for the surgery.

My Transformation

A week after my liposuction decision, I bumped into a friend I hadn't seen in a few years. She looked amazing. She was lean, toned, strong, and beautiful – exactly how I wanted to look. She referred me to her coach, whose first question was, *"What is your goal?"*

"I want to look like her," I answered while pointing to a fitness magazine cover model. Six months later, I achieved what I hadn't accomplished in two years – total body transformation. I looked and felt much better than I envisioned. Suffice it to say, liposuction never happened.

I became a different person – happy and confident, with a healthier mind, body, and a better circle of friends who shared similar goals. I also made more money because I was showing up more confidently and owning my brilliance.

My weight loss was primarily nutrition, but my journey stoked a burning desire to work out. Nicknamed *"G.I."* – for the character G.I. Jane – I went hard at the gym. With my weight loss goal achieved, I was excited and motivated to keep pushing. I went on to be a competitive bodybuilder, and I competed for four years. This led to my passion for helping women achieve the same physical, mental, spiritual, and life transformations I experienced. Fifteen years after my journey began and over 21,000 women's bodies transformed, I am committed to liberating women to step into their power and create happy outcomes.

Reading this book will give you exclusive access to my four-step weight loss system that will push you to lose weight while eating carbs and without drastic dieting or exercise. This book is the answer to your weight loss struggles and being overweight.

If you want to transform your body by losing from 10 to over one hundred pounds, enjoy shopping for clothes, and no longer dread getting on the scale at the doctor's office, then this book is for you.

While I can't promise you'll lose all your unwanted weight overnight, I can promise that your dress size will decrease through my step-by-step method to lose weight and feel great. And, if you follow the techniques I reveal in this book, it's highly possible you can enjoy the rest of your life unburdened by how you look. Don't wait until your anxiety gets the best of you, following your next social invitation to begin transforming your body. Get started on your weight loss journey today.

HELP! I'M OVERWEIGHT

CHAPTER 1

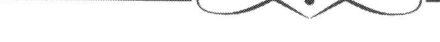

"Let food be thy medicine and medicine be thy food."
(Hippocrates, n.d.)

Lose Weight Without The Wait

CHAPTER 1

HELP! I'M OVERWEIGHT

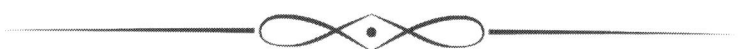

In your opinion, what does it mean to be overweight? I define being overweight as carrying excess weight or weighing more than the recommended amount. To those of us who've been overweight before, it means going up in clothes sizes, which sometimes means less variety of clothes, settling for stretch fabric with Spanx to hide the bulges or elastic jeans to prevent your stomach from getting a bruise from the imprint of the belt buckle.

Being overweight is a complex issue. It can negatively impact a person's physical and mental health and well-being. One of the most common issues associated with excess weight is a lack of confidence and self-love. Feeling unhappy with your body shape or size, can lead to feelings of inadequacy, low self-esteem, and even depression.

> *"Being just 10 pounds overweight increases the force on your knees by 30 to 40 pounds with every step you take."*
> (Fontaine, n.d. as cited in Jaret, 2019)

Being overweight puts extra strain on the body's organs, bones, and joints, leading to health complications like heart disease, stroke, diabetes, and joint pain. Additionally, carrying excess weight can make it challenging to move around and participate in physical activities, further contributing to weight gain and a sedentary lifestyle.

The physical and mental effects of being overweight can be overwhelming, along with determining the causes of being overweight in the first place.

My Complex Causes of Being Overweight

One of the leading causes of being overweight is consuming more calories than the body needs regardless if you are physically active or not. When a person consumes more calories than they burn, the extra energy is stored as fat. This may lead to weight gain and obesity over time.

I was overweight due to several reasons so there is no simple answer as to why. I had excess weight due to cultural and financial reasons, emotional and mental wellness, and lifestyle.

Culture & Emotional

I was born in Kenya in 1979. Growing up in Kenya, I was taught to view food as a privilege. Some families were not fortunate enough to have enough food, so we were introduced to eating everything on our plates and appreciating the meals we were given. At home, we ate mostly home-cooked food: chicken, rice, vegetables, and traditional Kenyan food, with a sprinkle of fast foods, usually as a treat after church or once a week. Portion control was not stressed.

From ages 13-18, I attended boarding school. The food at boarding school was nasty. However, we needed to eat all three meals, and of course, we had to clean our plates. I did what I was told and ate the food, but then I would binge at night on junk food.

In addition, at age 14, my parents separated and began going through a divorce. I was devastated because I was a daddy's girl who wanted to see her dad, but at the time, my mother didn't think it was best. I had to intervene in physical altercations between my parents and then cope with the emotional strain of their divorce.

The chaos at home led to me being diagnosed with migraines. This diagnosis caused me to eat even more junk food. Therapy wasn't an option with everything going on at home, and I didn't talk about how I felt. Eating was therapy. Therefore, at boarding school, I ate at night to ease the pain, which led me to being a very chubby teenager. By the time I was 15 years old, I weighed more than my mother and was often confused to be her sister.

Financial & Lifestyle

I went away to the United States for college because both my mother and I wanted me to have the best possibilities. I was 20 years old and my goal was to finish school, get a good job, and make a lot of money.

While in college, I worked two to three jobs, went to school full-time, and still had little money. I would eat at Wendy's because I worked there, or noodles and any other cheap and fast food. I took advantage of being in America because the food was inexpensive and no longer considered a privilege like in Kenya.

In America, I also had access to free food. At school, there would be free pizza. I remember attending the international student meetings. I would load up on free food and save some for later. I would eat one donut during the meeting and take one or two home that same day. I had no weight issues at this time because I was constantly moving around. My eating choices were not a priority. Thus, age and activity were on my side, although I only slept four to five hours a night.

I graduated college at age 25 and settled in Georgia because there was no snow, and I liked the weather. I got married at 26. He was American and from Louisiana. He was 14 years older than me, but he made me feel secure because he was financially stable. We enjoyed a lifestyle of travel, shopping, eating, partying, and having a good time.

My husband loved to spoil me with fine dining and four-course meals. We loved Sunday brunch because afterward, we would go home and take a nap.

I started gaining weight, but my husband always complimented me, so it didn't bother me. After we divorced, my weight was a problem because I didn't feel good about myself. This was the main reason for my determination to get rid of the unwanted weight.

After losing weight in 2010 and maintaining my healthy lifestyle for years, in 2017, I lost my only sibling, my brother, to suicide. This life event sent me spiraling out of control mentally and emotionally. As a result, I turned to stress eating. In two weeks I had gained 15 pounds!

From my experience, excess weight causes are complex and can change over time. Whatever the causes of your excess weight may be, it's essential to look at why you're struggling with weight gain in order to better address it.

There were various contributors to my weight gain. I've noticed it's been the same for my weight loss clients. Although there is no one reason for gaining weight, here are the common contributors for women over 40 being overweight.

Over 40 & Overweight
Busy Lifestyle

Many of my clients are women between the ages of 40-55. For women in this age group, focusing on weight loss can be a challenge. Between family, work, and other obligations, finding time and energy can be difficult. Women in this age group often juggle numerous responsibilities, such as family, pregnancy, career, and finances, all of which can lead to stress and emotional eating. Unfortunately, healthy habits often take a backseat during this time. Despite the difficulties, prioritizing health by incorporating healthy meal planning and other healthy habits into your lifestyle, can make all the difference.

Stress and Emotions

Food is a tool often used for emotional regulation. From celebratory events to sorrowful ones, we turn to food to fuel our emotions. Women over 40 commonly use food to feel happy or cope with sadness. When feeling stressed, the body sends out cortisol, also known as the stress hormone. Cortisol increases cravings for sugar, salty, and fatty foods because your brain thinks it needs fuel to fight whatever threat that is causing the stress even when this urge to eat isn't the result of an empty stomach Unfortunately, women who have experienced trauma like abuse or neglect may also turn to food for comfort, leading to emotional eating and weight gain. Furthermore, stress can disrupt sleep patterns, making it harder to regulate our appetite and metabolism.

Financial & Lifestyle

Financial concerns are another cause of being overweight. Those from humble beginnings may overeat when they achieve their financial goals. The amount of money plays a part because those with little funds eat cheaper foods. After all, money is scarce. The more affordable foods aren't the most nutritious and often contain many fats. Therefore, there is a positive correlation between little money and less healthy food causing weight gain.

On the contrary, those with a lot of money overindulge in food because they can. They identify success with "good food," which tends to be rich in price, texture, and calories. Portion size isn't considered because eating well feels good and symbolizes success for some women.

You are Overweight, so What are You Going to Do About it?

The cause of being overweight is overeating and moving less. This combination builds fat in the body, leading to confidence issues and self-love.

If you're like most women, then you've been on a never-ending quest to lose weight. You've tried every fad diet out there, only to find yourself back at square one a few weeks later. You're frustrated, and it's taking a toll on your self-confidence.

The problem is that most traditional weight loss methods are ineffective at best and downright dangerous at worst. Restrictive diets can lead to nutrient deficiencies and unhealthy obsessions with food, while harsh exercise regimens can cause injuries and lead to burnout.

I am here to provide you with a sustainable solution to lose weight without drastic dieting or exercise and keep the weight off for good. By following the simple steps in this book, you'll be on your way to your ideal weight in no time - without sacrificing your health or sanity.

Here are the reasons you are ready to lose weight without the wait:

1. **Happy & Healthy**: You want to be the life of the party. You are ready to be seen and heard and look forward to family events, socializing, dating, and being in all the pictures and not the picture taker. You will also live longer. You will reduce your chances of various health problems, such as heart disease, stroke, diabetes, and certain types of cancer. Studies have shown that losing weight can reduce your risk for these conditions and improve your overall health.

2. **Social & Emotional**: You will look forward to enjoying shopping sprees with your friends. No more shopping at the plus size stores or getting embarrassed when you hear, *"We don't have that in your size."*

3. **Purpose and Prosperity**: Waking up well-rested, happy, and energized will be your norm. You'll have a pep in your step, enjoy daily activities, beat that afternoon slump, and be super productive. Losing weight will help you feel more energized and motivated, allowing you to pursue your passions and goals more quickly. You will have more focus and clarity, and you will enjoy your life better!

4. **Maximizing your potential**: Losing weight can even help you increase your earning potential. Studies have shown that people who maintain a healthy weight tend to show up more, perform better, and be more engaged at work. You will have a positive attitude, feel in control of your future, and start to attract the right people and opportunities - your life is going to level up!
5. **Relationships**: Your spouse or partner will enjoy your new playful, flirtatious confidence, which will reignite intimacy, passion, and lead to a fulfilling relationship. You will be complimented and remembered as the woman they met and fell in love with many years ago.
6. **Confidence**. You will look comfortably in the mirror, appreciate and love the sexy person staring back, wondering what took you so long to get to this happy place!

Can you imagine the above benefits for yourself? After you reflect on the causes of your weight gain, whether emotional, financial, cultural, or a mixture, you can look forward to the life you want and set weight loss goals to achieve it. This will cause you to have a better love and appreciation for yourself and your body.

Are you ready to lose weight? Continue with me as you prepare to transform your body and be at your ideal weight for good. This book will not only help you get the desired results, but help you prevent the problem from reoccurring in the future. Trust me; you are in the right place. In the next chapter, I will break down the evolution of food so you can understand that the problem is not all your fault.

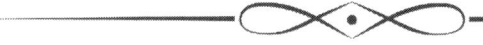

What's Eating You? What's Happening Now?

Chapter 2

"If nothing changes, nothing changes. If you keep doing what you're doing, you're going to keep getting what you're getting. You want change, make some."

(Stevens, n.d.)

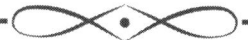

Lose Weight Without The Wait

Chapter 2

What's Eating You? What's Happening Now?

We went over the reasons that cause people to be overweight, but are you able to identify your reasons? Whenever we try to find answers to issues, we often start by addressing the root cause in order to pinpoint the problem. Have you ever done that when it comes to weight gain? Have you ever analyzed the history of why people are overweight?

Now if you are like me, then you could care less about the history of being overweight. You want to get straight to how you can lose weight for good. However, understanding the history of being overweight will help you see why so many are overweight and why obesity is such a problem. It also allows you to prevent making the same mistakes over and over again. Let's examine the history of the problem so you can conquer your weight now and keep it off in the future.

Weight Doctor

Do you ever wonder what goes on behind the scenes when you visit the doctor for a check-up? There's the paperwork, the measurements, and the analysis - all of which combine to determine what you need to live a long and healthy life. But what about when your check-up is for weight loss? While obesity isn't technically a "sickness," it significantly contributes to many health problems.

Why not treat it like a severe issue and seek professional help? Reading this book is your first step! Like a regular check-up, you work with a doctor. As your weight loss coach, I am here to help you tackle weight problems. Let's begin the process for a thinner, happier you!

Measurements

At the doctor, they measure our health by our blood pressure, and heart rate. What measurements do we use to measure our weight? Of course, it's the scale that we dread to step on, but BMI and WTH are other measurement tools.

BMI (Body Mass Index) and WTH (Waist-to-Hip) ratio are two standard measures used to assess body composition and the potential health risks associated with it.

The BMI ratio formula is your weight, (in kilograms) divided by height (in meters) squared. The resulting number falls into one of several categories: underweight (less than 18.5), average weight (18.5 to 24.9), overweight (25 to 29.9), or obese (30 or greater).

WTH ratio, on the other hand, is a measure of body fat distribution that compares the measurement and circumference of the waist to that of the hips. A high WTH ratio indicates that a person carries more fat around their waist, with a higher risk of developing health problems such as Type 2 diabetes, heart disease, and stroke. While BMI and WTH ratio are helpful indicators of body composition and health risks, they have different strengths.

BMI is a quick and easy measure widely used by healthcare professionals to screen for weight-related health risks. However, it does not consider body fat distribution, an essential factor in health risks. WTH ratio, on the other hand, provides information on body fat distribution and can help identify individuals who may be at higher risk of developing certain health conditions.

It is important to remember that no single measure can provide a complete picture of a person's health, and a comprehensive evaluation that includes other factors such as physical activity, diet, and medical history is necessary for a complete understanding of overall health.

In conclusion, BMI and WTH ratios can provide helpful information about a person's body composition and health risks. The choice of which measure to use depends on the specific needs and goals of the assessment.

Is Food The Problem?

Food has been a part of human history for as long as there have been humans. We have always had to find ways to get food by hunting, gathering, or growing it.

The way we get our food has changed a lot over time. *Hunter-Gatherer* culture was the way of life for early humans. The lifestyle of hunter-gatherers was based on hunting animals and foraging for food until 12,000 years ago when farming began. Then most people were farmers and they grew the food to feed their families. Today, only a tiny percentage of people grow their food. Most of us buy our food from grocery stores.

Food was created for nourishment, sustenance, and pleasure. It is a basic need of all humans and animals.

Nourishment is the most basic function of food. We need food to live. The nutrients in food give our bodies the energy and raw materials they need to function correctly. When we don't get enough nutrients, we become malnourished or even starve to death.

Sustenance refers to the continued provision of food over time. In other words, it is about sustaining life. When we talk about food sustenance, we are talking about having enough food to support ourselves and our families in the future.

Pleasure is another crucial reason we eat food. Food is one of life's great joys! Eating delicious foods can make us happy and help us bond with others. Sharing meals is also a vital part of many cultures around the world.

Consequently, food is essential for our survival. It gives us the energy we need to live and work; food also brings joy.

The Evolution Of Food Causing Obesity

The history of food is a long and fascinating story that tells us much about the human experience. From its humble beginnings as a means of survival to its current role as a source of pleasure and social interaction, food has always been an essential part of our lives.

History

The root of the problem of being overweight is complex and multifaceted, but one significant factor is the history of food and its evolution over time. Just like reviewing your family's medical history to evaluate yours, let's look at America's history with the consumption of food.

When looking at the history of food and being overweight, we can see that there have been drastic changes over time. Our diets changed from hunter- gatherers to the agricultural revolution then the industrial revolution, and then to the modern food industry. Here are some changes that led to the rise of obesity:

- » As agriculture developed, people started to cultivate crops and domesticate animals. This led to a more stable food supply and the consumption of more calorie-dense foods like grains and dairy products.

» Over time, food became easier to obtain and more affordable, leading to the rise of industrialization and the mass production of processed foods.
» The introduction of processed foods and abundant cheap, unhealthy food options made it easier to consume excess calories.

Today, many consume a diet high in processed foods, added sugars, and unhealthy fats, contributing to weight gain and other health problems. In addition, sedentary lifestyles and a lack of physical activity also play a significant role in the obesity epidemic. Obesity and weight gain have become a significant problem in our society today. Unfortunately, there is no single cause of obesity. Instead, it is caused by lifestyle habits and the amounts and types of foods we consume.

What are you eating?

If your blood pressure is too high when you go see the doctor, then a question they may ask is, what are you eating? Let's look at the food that can help to help improve your weight problem.

When it comes to weight loss, food is fuel. What you eat gives your body the energy to get through the day. Not all foods are created equal when it comes to weight loss. The key to successful weight loss is to focus on eating foods that will help you lose weight and avoid those that will make you gain weight. Foods that are high in nutrients and low in calories are ideal for weight loss.

Here are some examples of great weight-loss foods:

- » **Lean protein:** Lean protein helps build and maintain muscle mass, essential for burning calories and losing weight. Choose lean protein sources such as grilled chicken, fish, tofu, legumes, and eggs.
- » **Fruits and vegetables:** Fruits and vegetables are packed with fiber, vitamins, and minerals that support a healthy body. Plus, they're low in calories, making them a perfect weight-loss choice.
- » **Complex carbohydrates**: Complex carbohydrates give your body sustained energy throughout the day.
- » **Healthy fats:** Healthy fats like olive oil and avocados provide essential nutrients while helping you feel full and satisfied after meals.
- » **Low-fat dairy**: Dairy products are a great source of calcium, protein, and other essential nutrients. Choose low-fat varieties of milk, cheese, and yogurt.

Focusing on nutrient-dense, low-calorie foods can fuel your body, and you can healthily lose weight.

In addition to eating these healthy foods, you should drink plenty of water and limit your intake of sugary drinks, processed foods, and alcohol.

Exercise is also suitable for maintaining a healthy weight.

Exercise does the following for your body:

- » Improves flexibility, agility, and bone health.
- » Improves your memory and brain function, (all age groups).
- » Protects against many chronic diseases.
- » Lowers blood pressure and improves heart health.
- » Improves your quality of sleep.
- » Reduce feelings of anxiety and depression.
- » Combat cancer-related fatigue.

Please note exercise supports weight loss, but is not the primary cause of weight loss. Exercise and movement are great for overall health, but understand it is not a cause of the problem contributing to being overweight. No one is overweight because they do not exercise.

Remember that weight loss isn't about diet and exercise – it's about managing stress and emotions. If you're feeling overwhelmed or anxious, then try relaxation techniques such as yoga, meditation, or deep breathing. These can help you find inner peace and reduce the urge to comfort eat. You should identify patterns of behavior that lead to comfort eating. Once you're aware of these patterns, you can change them. For example, if you consistently eat when bored, find something else to do instead, take a walk, call a friend, or read a book.

Your Weight Loss Appointment Summary

To recap what we discussed earlier in this chapter, the reason so many are overweight is because the amount of food we consume has increased over time due to the following:

- » Accessibility: Food is easier to obtain; most people don't do physical work to get food.
- » Quantity: Food options have increased, providing us with more unhealthy options.
- » Availability: The usage of food has increased- making it not only a necessity but also a social and cultural enjoyment.

Understanding these factors and making healthy choices can help you maintain a healthy weight and prevent obesity-related diseases. Later in the book, you will see how this all works together in my four step proven weight loss method.

Lose Weight Without The Wait

Your Diet Failed...Again

Chapter 3

"When your brain is hooked on junk food, willpower, and personal responsibility don't stand a chance."
(Hyman, 2019)

Lose Weight Without The Wait

Chapter 3

Your Diet Failed...Again

What is your weight loss goal? Do you want to lose 20 or 50 pounds? More importantly, what's the reason you want to lose weight?

When people want to lose weight because they want to wear a bikini for the summer, then it is not a strong enough reason to help them to reach their goal. What do you see people posting on social media mid-spring? I'll go first, *"The summer is gonna get whatever body I give it."* That usually comes from people giving up on their goal of losing weight. They may take the approach, *"I will try again next year."*

What about the person who wants to lose weight to attend a high school reunion? They want to show off their credentials and prove that they have it going on, from their careers to how they kept their bodies up. What happens after the reunion? People resume the regular routines they had before they lost weight. Therefore, it is essential that your why is larger than the number on the scale to propel you forward and keep you from giving up or reverting to old habits.

What's Your Why?

Which scenario best describes you:

- » You feel embarrassed about your body and suffer from a lack of confidence and self-esteem.
- » You dread social settings and avoid pictures because you always seem to be the biggest person and feel judged based on how you look.
- » You suffer from mental fog and low energy hence doing the bare minimum at your job or business, missing out on promotions or business opportunities.
- » You secretly fear you will spend the rest of your life embarrassed miserable and ashamed of your body.
- » If you're single, you worry you won't ever find someone, or if you're in a relationship, then you fear your partner no longer finds you attractive.
- » You hide behind baggy stretchy clothes, girdles, or anything that will help enhance your appearance.

What's your reason for wanting to lose weight? Whatever your situation is, your emotions about your body may vary from others, but the one thing you have in common with other overweight women is you have tried to lose weight, but it didn't work!

Mind, Will, and Emotions

You know the saying you can do anything you put your mind to? I agree with it, and when it comes to losing weight, it is true. Your mind is potent, and you can use it for or against you in your weight loss journey, but it is all up to you.

You are in control! You control your body, and you control your mind. You determine if your mind will be a help to your body or a hindrance based on what you tell it. My goal is to help you use your mind to transform your body so that you can finally lose weight for good.

When I meet with new clients who want to lose weight, here is what I ask them:

- » What is your goal?
- » How much weight do you want to lose?
- » When was the last time you were at that weight?
- » How do you feel?
- » How do you perform your daily activities?
- » What changed since you were at your desired weight?
- » What are your habits? Do you drink wine every night? Eat dessert for lunch? What is your eating routine?

These questions are to help me understand what their struggles are contributing to weight gain to help them develop a sustainable goal and good reason why they want to lose weight.

As the prospects are answering the questions, frequently they can pinpoint how being overweight is affecting their daily lives. I've discovered that they did not have a good reason to lose weight before, which is the primary reason why they haven't lost weight.

As they start thinking about the questions to uncover, "the why behind the why," it encourages them to develop a more realistic goal for success. When they tell their mind that their weight loss is a short-term goal or quick fix, their mind and body will believe and follow that. On the contrary, when they develop the right reason to lose weight with a realistic time frame and plans to maintain the weight once they achieve their goal, their mind and body will comply with that also.

Plan To Succeed

You are probably thinking, what is a good reason to lose weight? Here are some of the whys from my successful clients versus the fad dieters.

Not-So-Good-Why: I want to lose weight to fit into my pre-pregnancy jeans.

Good Why: I gained weight during pregnancy, delivery, and breastfeeding. I want to get my weight down to have more energy for my children, increase intimacy with my husband, and perform my best at work and home.

Bingo! The goal above is good because it emphasizes tangible, long-term goals for losing weight versus superficial reasons like the other. A good goal will pass the test of time, (be ongoing), leading to a healthy mind, body, and lifestyle change.

Here Is Another Example:

Not-So-Good-Why: I want to wear a two-piece bathing suit to the beach next month.

Good Why: I want to feel comfortable in my clothes and my body and not dread when my kids ask me to go swimming.

The good why above is not short-term, it's sustainable for a lifestyle change versus a temporary fix.

Your Why

Take control of your weight loss journey by defining your goal. Like anything else, a weight loss goal has to make sense if you want to achieve it.

The S.M.A.R.T. goal method is great for financial purposes and for business goals. However, S.M.A.R.T. goals have proven successful for other objectives, so you should create them for your weight loss goal. Here are S.M.A.R.T. goals for weight loss below:

S- Specific: What is the specific amount of weight you want to lose, and how do you plan on losing it?

M- Measurable: How will you measure if you are doing the right things to lose weight? A weight loss scale, accountability, group, or professional program?

A-Achievable: Were you at this weight in the past? A goal within reach is realistic versus a weight you've never been at before.

R- Relevant: Your goal is based on a lifestyle change that will affect you ongoing versus just a short period.

T- Time: How long are you committed to achieving your weight loss goal based on the program length you choose?

Here is an example of a S.M.A.R.T. weight loss goal:

Specific- Lose 20 pounds through the ***P.U.S.H. System.***

Measurable- Weekly weigh-ins and check-ins with a coach and group meetings.

Achievable - You were at this weight before you had children. This goal is within reach.

Relevant - Achieving this goal will increase your confidence allowing you to show up more to grow your business.

Time - The course is six weeks and you will be able to maintain the weight loss over time.

A good weight loss goal incorporates your why. Your why will lead your mind and body to success. This brings great benefits! Your self-esteem and confidence will increase, you will feel better, and it will improve your relationships (and maybe even your work) in multiple ways.

Don't be the person who wants to lose weight to attend a high school reunion or another event. Because after the reunion, you will resume the routine you had before you lost weight.

Take control of your mind and body. Make sure "your why" is bigger than the number on the scale (your weight), and break down your weight loss goal the SMART way.

Lose Weight Without The Wait

Don't Do That, Do This!

Chapter 4

"90 percent of people who lose a lot of weight eventually regain just about all of it."
(Runge, n.d. as cited in Taylor Lippman, 2021)

Lose Weight Without The Wait

Chapter 4

Don't Do That, Do This!

You've tried and failed at every diet and exercise routine known to man. You've counted points and calories, cut carbs, fasted, and tried living on nothing but grapefruit, cabbage, or tomatoes. You've busted your butt at the gym—okay, okay, maybe not for a while. But you HAVE tried working out, and no amount of crunches EVER changed your waistline significantly.

You've attempted to accept your body the way it is ... but at the end of the day, your belly seriously impacts your body image. Does this sound like you? Trust me, I have been there! I tried **23** different diets and almost gave up until I found the solution to not only lose weight and keep it off, but also to feel great about my body.

Here are four weight loss mistakes that have kept people from reaching and maintaining their ideal weight:

1. Wrong Mindset

Our mindset can be a significant roadblock to successful weight loss. Believing that we are somehow "too old" or our genetics doom us to be overweight is not only untrue, but it keeps us from trying! It is possible to lose weight, no matter how old you are.

You need an empowering belief in yourself and determination - if you've tried everything without lasting success, then don't give up. It is not age, genetics, or any other factor that determines your success in weight loss. Your attitude and dedication can make all the difference in achieving your desired results. Staying positive can help you stay motivated throughout the process. Keeping this in mind, you can make sure that your mindset is working for you instead of against you. With the right attitude, anyone can achieve their weight loss goals!

2. Searching For Quick Fixes

Fad dieting is a quick fix to lose weight, but it is a mistake for sustainable weight loss. Many fad diets focus on extreme calorie restriction or eliminating entire food groups, which can be challenging to maintain over the long term.

Fad diets might seem fruitful initially, but they come with many drawbacks: relentless hunger pains, fatigue due to low-calorie intake, moodiness, and an unsustainable cycle, which often leads back to gaining the same pounds again.

Realizing weight loss isn't just about jump-starting your metabolism; rather true success lies in maintaining results through sustainable measures.

3. Relying on Exercise for Weight Loss

"You can't exercise your way out of a bad diet"
(Hyman, 2019)

Shedding unwanted pounds can be a daunting task, but understanding how the body uses energy is necessary to focus on the right approach. Some may think that exercise alone will do the trick - yet only 5% of your progress comes from exercise.

70% of calories are burned as the body performs basic life-sustaining functions like breathing, and blood circulation while you relax or sleep. This is known as your basal metabolic rate (BMR) or resting metabolic rate (RMR); an additional 15% of calories are burned for everything we do that is not sleeping, eating or sports-like exercise such as walking, taking stairs, vacuuming, doing the dishes, playing fetch with the dog, talking, standing, tapping your foot, cooking, yard work and so on and known as non-exercise activity thermogenesis (NEAT).

10 % of calories are burned through digesting and absorbing the nutrients from food. This is the thermic effect of food (TEF) and of all three food groups, protein, carbohydrates, and fat, protein requires the most energy to digest. Consequently, calories burned from any planned exercise is only 5% and is known as exercise activity thermogenesis (EAT). That's why exercising hard

without focusing on nutrition won't get you far in shedding extra kilos - as evidenced by my journey where I had trained extensively for two years with little results before finding out about proper eating habits.

When it boils down to what matters when trying to slim away those stubborn love handles - it's creating an environment in your body through diet adjustment that allows fat-burning mechanisms to take place, thus achieving the caloric deficit needed for the desired outcome.

4. Going at it alone

Weight loss is a goal shared by many, but it's not always successful due to lack of guidance and support. This multibillion dollar industry makes huge promises for instant results that rarely last in the long run. True transformation requires reprogramming our habits over extended periods - unlearning bad eating practices and learning sustainable lifestyle choices that guarantee success both now and later on.

I learned this lesson after two years of frustration, waiting time, energy, and financial losses caused by trying to go at weight loss alone, which almost led me down an even worse path with liposuction as the solution! Don't make the same mistake I was about to. The right information, guidance, and accountability to ensure you're heading towards your goal is your saving grace when it comes to achieving your target weight.

Busting Six Common Weight Loss Myths

While it can be challenging to shed those extra pounds, several common dieting myths may hinder your success. By understanding these errors and how to avoid them, you will soon be back on track to reaching your health goals. Here, I'll debunk the various myths so that you can apply what works.

Give up your favorite food to lose weight.

It's impossible to assume you will never have another glass of wine, a slice of pie, or cake because you are losing weight. This sets you up for failure and might increase cravings or binge eating. A good program or regimen accounts for or allows for enjoyment of everything in moderation.

Eating out is a no-no, and *all* food must be cooked at home.

Socializing and spending time with friends and family adds richness and texture to life; being unable to enjoy social activities can cause anxiety and develop a negative relationship with food.

Eat less, more like starving to lose weight.

It's the opposite. It would help if you ate (enough) to lose weight, unlike most drastic diets such as juicing, tomato soup, or cabbage soup diets that have you eliminate a lot of foods and starve the body, which might bring about fast weight loss and also fast weight gain once you resume normal eating.

Carbs are evil and are to be avoided.

The body depends on carbs for energy production. Unhealthy carbs are the problem and should be minimized, and the majority of carbs consumed should come from healthy options, as described later in this book.

Weight loss supplements are the answer to weight loss.

More effort is needed, and the only successful way to lose weight is by changing your nutrition habits.

If the scale is not moving, you are NOT making progress.

This is the easiest way to sabotage your efforts and cause you to throw in the towel. The scale is not the most accurate measure of progress. Non-Scale Victories (NSVs) are way more objective measures of progress than the scale, and here are eight common non-scale measures that you can begin to experience in as little as one week of eating the right way:

- » More energy and being able to accomplish more than usual
- » Better sleep and waking up refreshed
- » Clothes fitting looser
- » Skin improvement
- » Mental clarity and increased wellbeing
- » Reduced or eliminated knee and back aches
- » Lower blood pressure for those suffering from hypertension
- » Reduced glucose levels for Type 2 Diabetics

It's not easy to stick to a healthy diet and reach your goals. However, with the proper knowledge and outlook, you can overcome the obstacles that stand in your way. Never give up on yourself. You can achieve anything, starting by debunking all these health myths, and diet-related mistakes.

How My Clients Lose Weight

My approach to weight loss involves moderation through a nutrition plan that is simple to follow, flexible enough to allow for occasional indulgences, and sustainable for long-term success. If you want a foolproof method for success, then I highly recommend reading this book, which describes my unique *P.U.S.H. Weight Loss Method* to achieve your weight goals.

P.U.S.H. Method

I'm the creator of the *P.U.S.H. Weight Loss System* that focuses on nutrition changes because over 80% of weight or fat loss comes from nutrition changes. I created this weight loss system method because it is how I have maintained my ideal weight for over the last decade.

My goal is to reach 1,000,000 women to let them know that losing weight is possible and straightforward, especially using my P.U.S.H. Weight Loss Method. It's not about exercise, starvation, drastic diets, or misery. It's about respecting the power of food as good nutrition and wanting to fuel your body with the best quality/grade of fuel possible.

My ***P.U.S.H. Method*** helps busy, professional women between the ages of 35 and 75 to achieve body transformation by losing between 20 to 120+ pounds through nutrition. Without having to exercise so that they can fall in love with themselves, look great, feel fantastic, and lead a better, healthy, happy, and fulfilled life.

I only work with women ready to commit to doing what it takes to lose weight once and for all. Women who are action takers, coachable, and have a positive attitude. I reject clients looking for weight loss shortcuts or fads, do not take direction, and complain a lot. Without my help, these women continue to struggle with low self-esteem, lack of confidence, feeling invisible or judged by friends, low energy levels, and hiding from life.

This can make life a living hell because they feel uncomfortable in their skin. With my help, which you are getting from this book, women transform their bodies, feel sexy, regain confidence and control of their relationships, attract new friends, enjoy shopping for smaller, more stylish clothes, and become better versions of themselves. This benefits everything in their life because they will feel alive, empowered, re-energized, and enjoy a high quality of life.

With the ***P.U.S.H. Method***, you will be well on your way to seeing great results! Don't wait any longer; continue reading and reclaim control of your life for good!

Fuel For The Fire

Chapter 5

*"Every time you eat or drink,
you are either feeding disease or fighting it."*
(Morgan, n.d. as cited in Reier, 2018)

Lose Weight Without The Wait

Chapter 4

Fuel For The Fire

Are you fighting to stay alive, or do you continue eating poorly because your doctor hasn't diagnosed you with a debilitating disease "yet?" What will it take? A report from the doctor that tells you to eat healthily or die, or will you get sick and tired of being sick and tired?

Changing your eating habits can be a game-changer for your physical and mental well-being. Your body is an incredible machine that requires the right fuel to keep running smoothly. Unfortunately, most of us tend to fill it up with junk food and other unhealthy options, which can make us feel sluggish and tired all day long.

Are you ready to lose weight and feel great?

In this chapter, I am going to go over the first pillar of my *P.U.S.H. Weight Loss Method,* which is the **P, Purge unhealthy foods.**

Purge doesn't mean eating until you are full and then purging by putting your fingers down your throat to throw up the food you just ate. To purge means to stop eating unhealthy food altogether. Here's the good news: by eliminating these bad habits, you can not only meet your weight loss goals but also improve your overall longevity.

Breaking Down

Your body doesn't discriminate between types of food, but it knows how to break down everything you eat into its fundamental building blocks. Glucose, the product of digesting carbs, (and that irresistible cookie), is a crucial energy source for your cells. Meanwhile, protein - whether you prefer fish, chicken, or tofu - gets broken down into amino acids, which are essential for building tissues like skin, hair, and nails. And even though your taste buds have their preferences regarding fatty foods (hello, coconut oil), your body is just as adept at metabolizing different fatty acids.

Ultimately, all three of these building blocks - glucose, amino acids, and fatty acids - become the raw materials your body uses to keep moving along, from hormones to cells and everything in between. Thus, if you want the highest quality glowing skin, good hair, ageless features, and a flat stomach, then give your body the best quality fuel (food).

Premium Fuel

Your body is the ultimate machine, capable of extraordinary feats, but it requires fuel to function at its best. Just like you wouldn't expect a Honda to perform like a Ferrari on low-grade gas, you can't expect your body to function at its fullest potential on a diet lacking proper nutrients. Treat your body like the luxurious vehicles you dream of driving and fuel it with the highest quality "gas." Your body will thank you by performing at its best and serving you well for years.

Sometimes people come to me saying, *"I eat pretty healthy."* Still, after assessing, they realize what they think is healthy, isn't. The truth is, many of us think we eat pretty healthily, but when it comes down to it, we might not make the best choices. We might unknowingly sabotage ourselves with unhealthy food combinations or excessive portions.

It's time to face the facts and give our bodies the rest they deserve. To do that, we need to eliminate some of our favorite guilty pleasures—the ones that are our Achilles Heel, if you will.

Purge Unhealthy Food List

Bad News: Say goodbye to sugary sweets like cakes and cookies. Wheat-based products like pasta and bread need to go, too. And let's not forget about alcohol - any kind needs to be cut out. But it's not just the obvious culprits that need to be tossed. Greasy fried foods like fries and pizza? Yeah, those can't stick around, either. The same goes for savory, salty, and crunchy snacks like chips and pretzels. It might sound harsh, but cleansing these foods from our diets can help us lose weight, improve our health, and feel great. Let's give ourselves a fresh start and ditch those tempting treats for good.

The unhealthy foods we love, enjoy, and can never seem to get enough of, we have formed neural pathways in our brains that make them the automatic - go-to items when we're sad, happy, or stressed. Over time, they become what we eat without much thought or intention. We also have associated them with certain feelings, and the phrase, "comfort food," is an example of how we've attached our emotions to them. Moreover, these unhealthy foods become a part of our pleasure and reward system controlled by the brain.

Feel Good Food

Studies have proven that dopamine, the feel-good hormone, is released when your brain expects your favorite ice cream or chocolate bar. And after a stressful day or situation, the food of choice makes you 'feel better' even when the problem has not been solved or changed.

The continuous release of dopamine leads to a constant need to turn to ice cream or alcohol when you're stressed as a coping mechanism to make you feel better; however, it then turns into an addiction or coping mechanism.

Dopamine is the same hormone released when all drugs, sex, or gambling addicts chase 'the high' as higher quantities of dopamine are needed to achieve it. It's the same process with food and why people will suffer withdrawal symptoms from coffee, and sugar.

These same foods are the cause of disease. Case and point, cancer feeds on sugar. Type 2 Diabetes is a result of the body not being able to regulate glucose as a result of eating too many carbohydrates. Alzheimer's is now called Type 3 Diabetes because the very same glucose problem is wreaking havoc in the brain. Heart disease, the #1 killer, is a lifestyle condition caused by mismanagement of eating habits. Statistics show that, *"About 80% of chronic diseases are driven by lifestyle factors such as diet and exercise."* (Mladen Golubic,).

Purging Benefits

The unhealthy foods mentioned need to be purged to decrease inflammation in the body, which also decreases the risk of diseases. When you manage cravings caused by unhealthy foods, it activates and increases fat-burning for healthier food. It also reduces your appetite once the right foods are introduced, creating a caloric deficit needed for weight loss.

You can do anything you put your mind to. I know it's easier said than done, but once you decide to eliminate unhealthy foods, then you are on your way to your ideal weight and ideal life.

I usually say that nutrition for weight loss is like putting together a puzzle. It would help if you had all the pieces in the right places and in proper order to complete the puzzle correctly. If any one of the pieces are in the wrong place, then the puzzle won't fit. It's the same concept with weight loss, as you will discover as we walk through the other pieces…it won't work ;-)

Good news: The Purge phase is a way to reset your body. As previously mentioned, it's unrealistic to think you will never have a glass of wine or cookie because of your weight loss journey. The items purged can be reintroduced at a later time.

How To Properly Purge

Ready to kickstart your weight loss journey? Let's dive into the first pillar of my proven method: **Purging**. Follow these steps:

STEP 1: Take a good hard look at your diet and identify the unhealthy foods that seem to have a hold on you. You know the ones – the candy, the junk food, and the sugary drinks you can't resist. It's time to get real and make a list.

STEP 2: Find out why you like them or find them hard to eliminate. Dig deep to understand why you're so drawn to these foods. Does stress make you crave more sweets? Are you a comfort eater? Pinpointing the triggers will help you deal with them better.

STEP 3: Swap, swap, swap! Instead of unhealthy options, make healthier choices. Are you craving something sweet? Try a fruit smoothie. Need a savory snack? Go for some roasted nuts.

STEP 4: Knowledge is power. Educate yourself about the foods you eat – what's inside and their impact on your body. Knowing this will strengthen your resolve to stick to healthy options.

STEP 5: Integrate new healthy foods. Imagine how great it would feel if, only a few days into this course, junk food was entirely out of sight and out of mind! You can easily access healthy snacks every time hunger strikes - no more excuses or room for temptation as you take control of your eating habits.

Follow these five steps of the purging process, and you'll be amazed at how quickly your body responds to eliminating those unhealthy foods.

Let's say goodbye to unhealthy foods and drinks, and hello to a healthier, happier you! By purging your diet of junk, you can achieve weight loss and improve your overall health. But it's not just physical benefits that come with taking control of your nutrition; you'll also gain the confidence and energy you need to tackle life's challenges head-on! When you prioritize your health, you build a strong foundation for a better future, and by breaking free from unhealthy habits, you can develop a lifestyle that will support you for years to come. With determination and a commitment to healthy living, you can create an unstoppable you ready for anything life throws your way.

Reminder: Purging unhealthy foods is not something you will do forever, it is a temporary body reset and you can reintroduce the items in moderation later.

Lose Weight Without The Wait

First-class Body

Chapter 6

*"Your diet is a bank account.
Good food choices are good investments."*
(Frankel, n.d.)

Chapter 6

First-class Body

I believe everyone wants an upgrade. We decide to upgrade our cars when we reach a certain level of success, craving top-of-the-line quality and technology that surpasses our previous vehicle. We even splurge on seats offering more legroom and priority boarding on planes- after all, who doesn't want to feel like a VIP?

Upgrading isn't only reserved for material possessions; What about our food choices? If we truly desire a better lifestyle, then we must upgrade our eating habits. We can't keep consuming unhealthy food. It's time to level up and opt for better quality meals to help us achieve our weight loss goals.

Body Upgrade

When we consciously upgrade our food choices, we will feel physically and mentally better. The first step to attaining our weight goal is purging unhealthy food, as mentioned in the previous chapter. Additionally, the second pillar in my P.U.S.H. method is **U - Upgrading nutrition quality.**

Upgrading nutrition means eating foods closest to their natural form and source. It means eating foods from the farm, not factories, or processed plants. It's when you are eating foods in their natural state.

Upgrade

In the first step of our journey, we scratched the surface of how important raw materials are to creating and maintaining our bodies. Everything from our hair, to our skin, to our nails relies on a healthy and balanced diet. Surprisingly, even going skiing - yes, you read that right skiing - can benefit from better nutrition than processed foods.

By fueling ourselves with whole, natural foods, we give our bodies what they need to function optimally. Not only are these foods easily digested and eliminated, but they also provide us with ample energy to tackle our daily tasks, including complicated tasks such as skiing. Plus, they can help manage blood sugar levels, regulate cholesterol, lower blood pressure, and help us live longer and happier. Talk about a powerful punch! All these amazing benefits and non-scale victories (NSVs) make shedding weight a bonus or perk. Why not try whole foods and see their incredible impact on your health and well-being?

How To Upgrade Your Nutrition

Weight loss and good health follow good nutrition.

Many people do not eat healthy because they lack nutrition education. Food is divided into two groups: Macros & Micros.

Macros is short for macronutrients. Macro means significant, so macronutrients are the nutrients that your body needs in large amounts. There are three macronutrients: carbohydrates, protein, and fat.

Carbohydrates

Carbohydrates provide four calories per gram and are the primary source of energy for the body.

Carbs are the most misunderstood macronutrient. It's also the most abused and over-consumed one, and that leads to a lot of issues due to lack of education.

Carbs are divided into three groups:

1. Simple carbs
2. Complex or starchy carbs
3. Fibrous carbs

To better explain this, I'll use a dating analogy.

1. Simple carbs – "AKA" Easy Esther

The first carbohydrates for you to be aware of are simple carbs. "Simple" carbohydrates require little effort to break down into glucose, which is the body's primary fuel. They have a straightforward molecular structure, and once consumed, conversion to glucose is rapid and precise without much effort.

Easy Esther is down for whatever, she's the kind of girl who doesn't take much convincing from a guy to have sex on the first night.

Simple carbohydrates, also on their own as processed carbs, are similar to Easy Esther, with minimal processing effort needed. They are usually not in their natural form due to some alteration or processing in a mill. After consumption of simple carbohydrates, they are speedy to digest and provide quick energy.

This quick digestion and energy is because of a spike in glucose levels in the blood, which requires the liver to produce insulin, also known as the fat-storage hormone, to regulate. Once insulin is released, all-natural fat-burning stops.

Ever wonder why kids bounce off the walls 20 mins after eating a lot of candy, followed by a crash? That's because of a glucose spike from eating a lot of simple sugars.

Simple carbs include cake, cookies, sodas, ice cream, donuts, and cocktails. Some fruits, those with a high glycemic index, fall under this category, too because of sugar/sweetness. However, simple carbs aren't always sweet foods. Certain foods are not sweet but are fast to digest and spike glucose levels. These include bread, pasta, bagels, and croissants, usually made from processed wheat.

Rule of thumb: Simple carbs should be consumed in moderation because they are loaded with a lot of extra calories and devoid of nutrition

2. Starchy carbs/Complex carbs- AKA Hard to get Helen

The second carbohydrate group for you to gain clarity on is starchy carbohydrates, which are the same as complex carbs. The body requires a lot of energy and time to digest and absorb complex carbs because they have complex molecular chains, and a lot of energy/calories are needed to break the food down. They take a longer time to digest, and for this reason, glucose is absorbed into the body at a slower rate compared to simple carbs.

Hard to Get Helen; as the name suggests is complex. She requires effort from a man she's dating and might have a six-month rule before ever giving it up.

Examples of complex carbs: Sweet potatoes, quinoa, buckwheat, and oats.

Rule of thumb: Starchy or complex carbs are healthy and provide a clean energy source, unlike simple carbs.

3. Fibrous Carbohydrates –"AKA" Gracious Grace

The third carbohydrate group is fibrous carbs. Fibrous carbs, or vegetables, require the most effort to break down or digest because they have fiber/roughage thanks to cellulose. They also have what simple & starchy carbs lack besides fiber, lots of much-needed or essential vitamins and minerals but low in energy and calories.

Gracious Grace is a good girl. Her dating rule is simple: the cookie stays in the cookie jar, aka no sex before marriage.

THINK GREEN.

Examples of fibrous carbs are cauliflower, kale, broccoli, and spinach. The type of carbohydrates in veggies is NOT the same in starchy carbs.

Rule of thumb: Vegetables are rich in much-needed vitamins and minerals that other foods do not have. They fill us up quicker, keep us full longer, and are low in calories.

Not all Carbs are Created Equal

It's time to discover the surprising truth about losing weight while satisfying your carb cravings! It's possible to shed those extra pounds even while enjoying the energy-boosting benefits of carbohydrates. However, not all carbs are the same, and simply cutting back on processed foods won't cut it. Instead, focus on incorporating more starchy and fibrous carbs into your diet while minimizing simple carbs. You'll be amazed at how delicious and satisfying these healthy carb options can be!

Carbohydrates Recap For Weight Loss

Don't swear off carbohydrates yet. You can use these macros to support your weight loss goals by making wise choices. First, the easy, (but not-so-healthy) option: is processed carbs. *Easy Esther*'s a fan, but if you hope to slim down, you'll want to cut back on these empty calories. Next, we've got starchy carbs, which are a bit harder to digest, but pack a nutritional punch, providing your body with energy and nutrients. *Hard to Get Helen*'s a toughie, but consuming this type of carb in moderation is vital to losing weight.

Finally, we have the fibrous carbs, AKA vegetables. These are the reigning champs of the carb world, although they require more effort to digest. *Grace* may be gracious, but she's not messing around regarding delivering nutrients and supporting weight loss. There you have it - a brief rundown on how to work with carbs to achieve your fitness goals.

In conclusion, it's crucial to stay away from processed foods, which the food manufacturers keep you indulging in.

The *P.U.S.H. Method* is a great tool to lose weight and feel great for good. Remember, while carbs are essential, it's important to remember not all carbs are made equal. Complex carbs in moderation should always be the main focus when choosing meals, snacks, and treats. Add in some fibrous options, and you're well on your way to reaching your health and fitness goals. In the following

Lose Weight Without The Wait

chapter, we'll learn about how protein and fats are essential aspects of this journey as well. Strap on that seatbelt because it's time to go deeper in your weight-loss adventure with the P.U.S.H. Method!

Body Upgrade

Chapter 7

"Food is not just fuel. Food is about family, food is about community, food is about identity. And we nourish all those things when we eat well."
(Pollan, n.d.)

Lose Weight Without The Wait

Chapter 7

Body Upgrade

Imagine your body was a luxurious Bentley or Maserati; would you settle for low-grade fuel? Of course not!

You deserve the best fuel for your beautiful machine - the same goes for your body. Just as high-quality gas is essential for premium cars, nutritious food is vital for our bodies. Don't settle for cheap, unhealthy food when you can nourish yourself with the best nutrition available. Remember, you're more than a car, and you deserve top-quality care.

Many of us can be incredibly tenacious in reaching our educational, work, and financial aspirations. Yet, when it comes to losing weight and maintaining our ideal weight, we often see a fluctuation on the scale. Emotional reasons and other chaotic life events can cause this, but we do not give up on our careers despite any obstacles. We power through them.

Similarly, we can tackle our weight loss goals with the same determination for everything else within our control. The same way we choose to succeed in our professions is how we can prefer better nutrition habits that can help us achieve our weight goal.

Step 2: Upgrading Your Food

As discussed in the previous chapter, the second part of my P.U.S.H. Method is upgrading your food's quality. We discussed how to upgrade while eating more complex carbs and vegetables. Now let's discuss the other two parts of the macronutrients to lose weight, which are protein and fats.

Protein - How to lose weight eating protein

Think of protein as a superhero for your body. It's the one that does all the heavy lifting inside your cells and keeps everything running smoothly. Without it, your body wouldn't be able to function correctly. Protein is not just any ordinary nutrient; it's the backbone that supports the structure, function, and regulation of all your body's tissues and organs.

Protein provides four calories per gram and is found throughout the body—in muscle, bone, skin, and hair. It makes up the enzymes that power many chemical reactions and the hemoglobin that carries oxygen in your blood. At least 10,000 proteins make you what you are and keep you that way.

Proteins are made up of building blocks called amino acids. There are about 20 different amino acids that link together in various combinations. Your body uses them to make new proteins, such as muscle and bone, and other compounds, such as enzymes and hormones. It can also use them as an energy source.

The top two primary protein sources are animal and plant-based protein.

Animal protein - Animal protein offers a wide variety of options, including meat like chicken, beef, and lamb, fish and seafood, eggs, and yogurt.

1. **Plant-based sources** include - tofu and tempeh, made from soybeans, provide a healthy and eco-friendly alternative.

Did you know beans and lentils have more carbs than protein? They have higher amounts of protein than most VEGETABLES, but they have three times as many carbohydrates. This is the same for quinoa. If you compare rice or other carbs to quinoa, quinoa has a bit more protein, but it really should be considered a carbohydrate.

Rule of thumb: Animal protein sources should have minimal visible fat. Choose lean cuts of beef for weight loss.

Fats

We went over protein and carbohydrates. Fats are the third component of macronutrients. Fats are essential for how your body uses many vitamins and plays a role in how all cells in the body are made and work.

Dietary fat provides nine calories per gram and comes from food. The body breaks down dietary fats into fatty acids to make the fats it needs. But all dietary fats are not the same. They have different effects on the body. Some dietary fats are essential. Some increase the risk for disease, and some help prevent disease.

There are two main kinds of dietary fats: saturated and unsaturated fat.

1. Saturated fats

Saturated fats are usually solid at room temperature and can visibly be seen on certain products.

Foods high in saturated fats include:

- » Meats, including beef, lamb, pork, and poultry, especially with skin.
- » Lard, and Dairy products like butter and cream.
- » Whole-milk cheese or yogurt.

Saturated fat tends to raise levels of cholesterol in the blood. Low-density lipoprotein (LDL) is called "bad" cholesterol. High-density lipoprotein (HDL) is called "good" cholesterol. Saturated fats raise the levels of both.

The *Dietary Guidelines for Americans* suggest that less than 10% of calories a day should be from saturated fats. The American Heart Association recommends a goal of 5% to 6% of daily calories from saturated fats.

2. Unsaturated fats (Healthiest)

Unsaturated fats are usually liquid at room temperature and are good for you. There are two types of unsaturated fats, monounsaturated and polyunsaturated.

  a) **Monounsaturated fats** are good fats in avocados, almonds, cashews, peanuts, olives, and seeds (sunflower, flax). Cooking oils are made from plants or seeds such as sunflower, canola, soybean, olive, sesame, and peanut oils.

  b) **Polyunsaturated fats** are found in fish, sesame seeds, pine nuts, and Brazilian nuts. Polyunsaturated fats contain healthy omega 3 and 6 in fish, sesame, flaxseed, and chia seeds.

Despite unsaturated fats being healthy, they MUST be consumed in moderation because they are incredibly high in calories. For example

1 tbsp of olive oil = 120 calories

18g/18 pieces of almonds or 18g = 100 calories

18g/14 pieces of cashews or 18g = 100 calories

17g/2 tbsp of peanuts = 100 calories

18g/28 pieces of raw pistachios = 100 calories

100g/1/3 of a medium-sized avocado that should weigh about = 160 calories

32g/1 tbsp of natural peanut butter = 90 calories

Rule of thumb: You should eat 1-2 fats each day. Moderation is vital because small quantities of fat are dense in calories and despite having healthy sources, they will contribute to weight gain when over-consumed.

Eating Recap

We went over the three macronutrients. To upgrade your quality of food, focus on eating whole and natural foods

Examples:

Carbohydrates: Sweet Potatoes, Yams, Potatoes, Rice, Weetabix, Grits, Porridge, Carrots, beans, Peas, Lentils, Weetabix

Protein: Chicken, Fish & Seafood, Beef, Lamb, Eggs

Vegetables: Broccoli, Green beans/french beans, Spinach, Kale, Cabbage, traditional greens, Cauliflower, Bok Choy

Minimize caffeine - coffee & tea. Drink enough water. Here is a quick method to ensure you are drinking adequate water.

Water Intake: Your water intake should be based on how much you weigh.

<u>In Pounds and Ounces:</u> Your weight in pounds divided by 2= number of water needed in ounces.

<u>In Kilos and Liters:</u> Your weight in Kilos divided by 30= number of water needed in liters.

How to Upgrade To Lose Weight

Understanding food combinations is essential, and as the saying goes, *"Eat breakfast like a king, lunch like a prince, and dinner like a pauper."* This means the heaviest meal at breakfast, a good one at lunch, and a light meal at dinner. Here is how I recommend the macros combinations for different meals:

- » Breakfast - carbs + protein - vegetables are optional
- » Lunch - carbs + protein + vegetables
- » Dinner - protein & vegetables.

Eat most of your calories earlier in the day to prevent cravings and overeating at night time, which is a contributor to weight gain. Also, you should consume 80% whole and natural food sources while allowing 20% to enjoy treats or processed items in moderation for a healthy balance and to minimize feeling deprived.

Micronutrients

We reviewed the macronutrients (carbohydrates, proteins, fats) our bodies require in larger doses to perform at an optimum level. Now, let's get into the second thing our bodies need, micronutrients.

Micronutrients are nutrients that are required by the body in lesser amounts for its growth and development. They include vitamins and minerals vital to healthy development, disease prevention, and well-being. Except for Vitamin D, micronutrients are not produced in the body and must be derived from the diet.

Since our body cannot produce vitamins and minerals, they are taken externally from different food products. The micronutrient content of every food is different; therefore, it is advisable to eat varieties of food for enough vitamin and mineral consumption.

Micronutrients consist of 13 essential vitamins, which the body requires in small quantities every day. The importance of these vitamins cannot be underestimated. The 13 vitamins are A, C, D, E, K, and 8 B vitamins - thiamine, riboflavin, niacin, pantothenic acid, biotin, B6, B12, and folate.

Minerals - There are a lot, but 15 minerals are essential for health: calcium, phosphorus, potassium, sodium, chloride, magnesium, iron, zinc, iodine, sulfur, cobalt, copper, fluoride, manganese, and selenium. The minerals along with the vitamins are essential for health. If you are following my recommended tips in my weight loss method, then you should be receiving the right amount of vitamins and minerals you need.

Here is a chart of our upgraded food list for your convenience.

Protein	Vegetables	Carbohydrates	Fruit	Fats
Steak	Spinach	Red potatoes	Grapefruit	Coconut oil
Chicken breast	Broccoli	Sweet potatoes	Green Apples	Olive oil (uncooked)
Turkey	Asparagus	Squash	Watermelon	Avocadoes
Lean ground turkey/chicken/beef	Green beans	Rice	Cantaloupe	Nuts
Egg whites	Peppers	Pumpkin	Honeydew	
Tilapia	Kale	Yam	Strawberries	
Cod	Spinach	Butternut scotch	Blueberries	
Orange Roughy	Cabbage	Quinoa		
Halibut	Collard Greens	Oatmeal		
Grouper	Romaine Lettuce	Yucca		
Trout	Spring Mix			
Scallops	Cucumbers			
Cornish Hen	Zucchini			
Bison	Cauliflower			
Sea Bass	Brussel Sprouts			
Mushrooms				
Whey Protein				

In conclusion, the choice to upgrade our diets and embrace whole-natural foods is undeniably one of the best decisions we can make for our bodies. By opting for nutritious, wholesome options over processed foods, we take control of our health and lose weight. This step in my weight loss method will help ensure you lose weight. In the next chapter, we will go over the next phase of my weight loss method so keep reading!

Structured Eating

Chapter 8

"Healthy eating is a way of life, so it's important to establish routines that are simple, realistically, and ultimately livable."
(Horace, n.d.)

Lose Weight Without The Wait

CHAPTER 8

STRUCTURED EATING

Are you a mom struggling to shed those last few pounds? Maybe you've been trying different diets and programs, but nothing works. If that's your experience, then it could be time to change your approach and focus on scheduling when you eat.

In the previous chapters, we discussed what you should and shouldn't eat. Now it's time to focus on when you should eat and how. The third step in my P.U.S.H. Weight Loss Method is *S-Structure Your Food.*

The body loves structure. It loves predictability.

Imagine you just had surgery or are not feeling well. You get prescription medication from a doctor, with instructions, such as, "Take this three times a day with food." Some might even have said to take "Every 6 hours." If you miss the medicine at the prescribed time, then you begin to feel pain or become unwell, and your body quickly reminds you that you missed a dose. That is an example of medication timing at work.

The body is GREAT at remembering all the details, especially schedules.

Structuring your food is important because it can help make sure that your body has enough energy throughout the day while cutting out unhealthy snacks. In this chapter, we'll discuss how proper meal timing can optimize weight loss in busy women, even with hectic schedules.

Step 3: Structure Your Meals

Structured eating is an essential factor when losing weight. Our bodies are finely-tuned machines with a knack for consistency. An effective eating plan relies on setting a regular schedule. For example, newborn babies are known to keep new moms up the first couple of months by breastfeeding every three hours like clockwork. Who created their feeding schedule? How do they know to wake up crying every three hours for mom's milk? Eating on a schedule is ideal for their proper development so they prompt mothers at eating time. Unfortunately, once they reach a certain age, they get 'domesticated' or trained/acclimated to society's eating clock and adjust to its new schedule.

While structured eating is best for babies it's also best for you. Sporadic mealtimes may delay your best results and lead you away from achieving those health goals, so eating on a schedule is critical.

Structured eating involves planning and thinking about how much food you will consume in a day and when you will eat it. Structured eating helps your body to adapt to nutrition timing, which helps to maximize energy throughout the day.

Don't Make These Mistakes

Structuring your food means creating an eating schedule and sticking to it. Here are some examples of what random eating might look like:

Eating when you feel like it and what you feel like.

Eating twice a day some days, three over the weekend.

Drinking a lot of coffee throughout the day and eating once a day because you're never hungry yet wonder why you still gain weight or why you never lose weight.

Grazing throughout the day on light snacks or very light meals, and some days more than others.

All four above have one thing in common - no structure and lack of nutrition timing. Your body can barely anticipate what to expect on any given day. Some days you hardly eat enough; others, you overeat.

Lastly, think about your sleeping patterns. If you go to bed at a good time and the alarm goes off at six am every morning, chances are you stir a few minutes before or find yourself up at six am, even on Sundays when you don't have to wake up early.

Now imagine that you got a new job, and due to a longer commute, you must wake up at five am. The first week will be rough because your body is not used to being up that early. By the 3rd week, however, your body will stir right before the alarm at five am.

This is the structure that the body loves; you repeat an activity every day over and over, which leads to the automation of the process. Our bodies are amazing machines that love to watch and learn our patterns, then rise to meet us by trying to make the routine simpler, hence the word automation.

This automation happens in the brain by forming new neural pathways that simplify tasks the more we repeat them. This is the same case where nutrition is concerned. If you drink a lot of soda and not much water, then your neural pathway for drinking soda is automated and habitual. When you decide to ditch extra sugar, including soda, and drink water instead, it feels challenging at first. Still, as you keep drinking more water day in and day out, you will realize that it gets easier as the soda neural pathway gets weaker and the water gets stronger.

If you keep this up for a few months, then you will realize that you used to drink a lot of soda, and now you drink more water. Thanks to repetition, the neural water pathway takes over from the soda, and yes, a new habit is formed.

Eating at the same time every single day has a lot of great benefits, including:

- » The body can anticipate nutrition
- » It reduces your appetite, and the body adapts to the eating schedule
- » It eliminates idle eating
- » It promotes intentionally eating since you don't eat on a whim

How to Schedule Eating

- » Select a time to have breakfast daily, Monday to Friday, or all 7 days if possible.
- » Allow times in between meals and snacks or no eating to allow the body to fully digest and absorb the meal.
- » Between breakfast & lunchtime, allow a four-hour duration between the two. I call this the power of four hours, which is from one main meal to another.
- » If you prefer to have a snack between breakfast and lunch, then allow a three-hour duration between the two. This is the power of three hours between a meal and a snack or from a snack to a meal.
- » After lunch, you can choose to have a snack three hours later, or you can have dinner four hours later.
- » If your weekend starts later than a weekday, then create a weekend eating schedule.

What a Scheduled Menu Looks Like

Here is an example of what your scheduled meals would look like:

8 am: Eggs & Oats

12 pm: Chicken, Sweet potato & Spinach

3 pm: Apple

6 pm: Salmon and Green beans

OR

8 am: Eggs & Oats

11 am: Yogurt

2 pm: Chicken, Sweet Potato & Spinach

5 pm: Apple

8 pm: Salmon and Green beans

With structured eating, I also need to point out that portion control must be adhered to. It is possible to eat the right kinds of whole and natural foods and still gain weight from consuming huge portions.

Scheduled Sleep

Another thing you want to schedule is sleep. Although we multitask daily and still have items left on our to-do list, 7-9 hours is best for weight loss. Studies show that women who sleep five hours a night compared to seven weigh more, increase more over time, and are more likely to become obese.

In addition, one study shows that "Inadequate sleep:

Interferes with the body's ability to metabolize carbohydrates and causes high blood levels of glucose, which leads to higher insulin levels and greater body-fat storage.

Drives down leptin levels, which causes the body to crave carbohydrates.

Reduces levels of growth hormone- a protein that helps regulate the body's proportions of fat and muscle.

Can lead to insulin resistance and contribute to increased risk of diabetes.

Can increase blood pressure.

Can increase the risk of heart disease." (Shomon, 2023)

Therefore, schedule your sleep and be consistent with it to optimize your weight loss.

How To Manage Portion Controls To Lose Weight

Another thing to watch out for in addition to getting enough rest is how much you are eating. Here are two easy ways to manage portions:

The Plate Method

I am using a round plate and a lunch meal as an example. Let half of it be covered with vegetables, a quarter of carbohydrates, and quartered protein as an example of a meal.

The Hand Method

Protein should be the size of the palm of your hand, carbohydrates the size of your fist, and vegetables should be two handfuls.

Step 3 Summary

Scheduling your meals is an essential factor to consider when losing weight. Eating at regular intervals throughout the day will help you avoid overeating, stay full, and maintain consistent energy levels. Additionally, it can help regulate your metabolism and encourage healthy eating habits.

When scheduling meals for weight loss, it is vital to plan and consider your daily routine. If you have a busy day planned, then it may be helpful to pack snacks and meals that are easy to eat on the go or have them readily available at home. For example, if you're going out for lunch or dinner, then choose healthier options like a salad with grilled chicken instead of fried foods.

To achieve your weight loss goals, you must allow time to create an eating schedule to stay on task. Sometimes, I block off time on my calendar for my meals. By this, my other appointments won't interfere with me fueling my body. We set the alarm to remind us of upcoming meetings. Why not put the warning on when it is time to eat? After all, what is more important than taking care of your health?

Lose Weight Without The Wait

The Best Hack Ever

Chapter 9

*"I've been on a diet for two weeks
and all I've lost is two weeks."*
(Totie Fields, n.d.)

CHAPTER 9

THE BEST HACK EVER

―――――∞・∞―――――

Do you ever wonder why you stop losing weight while on a diet? Ever wonder why your weight reaches a standstill?

When you follow a weight loss routine for some time, you will eventually notice that the results have plateaued because your body will adapt to your current habits. To prevent this from stopping the pounds from falling off, you must keep your body challenged and continue toward weight loss success.

This chapter is the final step in my P.U.S.H Weight Loss Method. We discussed the foods to eliminate, what to add, and how to schedule meals to lose weight. Our final step is learning to *H-Hack Your Metabolism* to increase weight loss.

Hack Your Metabolism

Our bodies have a remarkable capacity for adapting and learning. While this is incredibly advantageous, as discussed in the previous chapter for *S-Schedule Structured Meals,* it also can become detrimental when you have more weight to lose, but your body has reached a standstill.

When losing weight, it's normal to lose weight when you first begin a new regimen and then notice that the progress starts to slow down as the body adapts or hits a plateau, which is also known as metabolic adaptation.

Metabolic adaptation is designed for our body's survival when faced with significant weight loss. Metabolic adaptation happens when our body adjusts to reduce our resting metabolic rate (RMR) to ensure we have enough fuel. By reducing our resting metabolic rate (RMR), this helps the body maintain its energy balance. The reason metabolic adaptation causes our weight loss to plateau is that during this time, our metabolism slows down to reduce the rate at which energy (calories) is burned. Therefore, our resting metabolic rate lowers to ensure we still have enough fuel to keep going!

The RMR is how many calories our body needs to function correctly and maintain weight, explained Caroline West Passerrello, MS, RDN, LDN, a spokesperson for the Academy of Nutrition and Dietetics. Consequently, once we lose a certain amount of weight, we need to hack our bodies to speed back up our resting metabolic rate leading to more weight loss.

How Do You Keep Losing Weight

After our bodies get accustomed to a new eating plan, weight loss will reach an equilibrium - that's your cue to switch up your routine and hack your metabolism successfully! Hitting a plateau can be extremely frustrating as you continue to eat healthily, but notice that the inches and scale have stopped moving. This means that it's time to change things up.

Hacking the metabolism doesn't mean reverting to unhealthy habits; it is all about diversifying your diet. In the world of exercise or fitness, you'll constantly hear, *"Change things up to keep your body guessing."* If you lift the same weight or run the same distance, the body adapts and progresses or gains a plateau.

To keep making gains, weights have to increase or the running intensity or distance have to increase. It's a similar concept with nutrition. Once your body is used to a certain nutrition regime, to keep losing weight your calorie intake has to change.

At this point, it is time to reassess your diet and lifestyle habits and make adjustments accordingly. You may need to adjust your calorie intake or switch up the types of foods that you are eating on a regular basis.

In addition, make sure to stay motivated and remain focused on your goals. Remember that no matter how slow the progress may seem, it is still progress and that is what really matters.

Here is what I find works best for my clients to hack their metabolism.

- » Eating foods that are in season since naturally not all foods are fresh in every season. This changes the normal food choices.
- » Reduce the amount of animal products such as chicken, beef, and fish and focus on plant based foods. A good way to do this is deciding to have one plant based meal a day or even take one week away from animal protein and instead eat more beans, lentils, and tofu.
- » Incorporate more additional healthy fats such as olives, avocado, and chia seeds.
- » Reduce the amounts of starchy carbs consumed with every meal.
- » Carb cycle - have days or weeks you're eating more carbs than others. For example, in the winter, comfort foods are a go-to for some, so these might be a few months with a bit more carbs in your diet than in the summer when it's easier for some to eat less carbs, drink more water, and eat more raw vegetables instead of cooked.

The goal is to keep the body challenged…guessing. Don't revert to old eating habits. Your body will go back to losing weight once you figure out the hack that works.

What will be your hack? There is no easy answer because everybody's food likes and dislikes are different. The key is enjoying a wide variety of foods and keeping an open or adventurous palate.

After you assess your diet and the foods you eat, see what options you can switch to that will give the same nutrition but still hack the body to keep losing weight.

Lose Weight Without The Wait

Weight Loss Method Final Notes

Chapter 10

"The distance between who I am and who I want to be is only separated by what I do!"— (Motivation Power, 2016)

Chapter 10

Weight Loss Method Final Notes

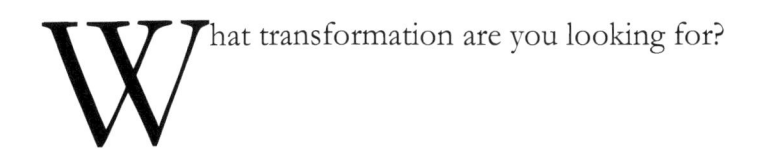

What transformation are you looking for?

- » Are you ready to finally stop yo-yo dieting and have a solution that works, and is sustainable?
- » Are you ready to rock your old smaller clothes without Spanx or other body products, and enjoy shopping again?
- » Are you ready to enjoy dating, hanging out with friends and family, and taking happy selfies?
- » Are you ready to wake up feeling energized, have a great day at work, play with your children and reignite your sex life?

If you are ready to finally feel comfortable in your own skin, then my proven weight loss system is for you. With over 668,615+ lives impacted online, 21,000+ transformations, and 7826+ nutrition plans to date, I created the P.U.S.H. Weight Loss Method to help end the fad diets, strenuous exercise routines, and every diet mistake or myth in between. Here is a summary of my four part weight loss system discussed in this book. See the summary below.

P.U.S.H.

Step 1: P - Purge unhealthy foods

Eliminate unhealthy foods.

Action:

Eliminate all processed and highly inflammatory foods for three weeks after which you can re-introduce treats in moderation.

How to implement:

Foods to eliminate-

- » Alcohol
- » Wheat products
- » Bread/croissants/bread/cookies/cake
- » Fried Foods - burgers, fries, pizza
- » Other junk - chocolate, sweets, ice cream, granola
- » Unhealthy drinks - juice, lattes, fruit smoothies, energy drinks

Step 2: U - Upgrade quality of foods

Action

Focus on eating whole and natural foods.

How to implement:

Foods to eat-

Carbohydrates: sweet potatoes, yams, potatoes, rice, grits, porridge, carrots, beans, peas, lentils.

Protein: Animal Based: Chicken, Fish & seafood, beef, lamb, eggs. Plant Based: beans, lentils, and tofu.

Vegetables: Broccoli, green beans/french beans, spinach, kale, cabbage, traditional greens, cauliflower, bok choy

Minimize caffeine - coffee & tea

Water: Drink enough water. Your water intake should be based on how much you weigh. Use this formula to calculate how much water to drink based on your weight.

<u>In Pounds and Ounces:</u> Your weight in pounds divided by 2= amount of water in ounces.

<u>In Kilos and Liters:</u> Your weight in Kilos divided by 30= amount of water in liters.

Snack: A snack should be no more than 200 calories. Healthy snacks should be readily available and simple to pack or carry. Here are some great options:

- Nuts: peanuts, almonds, cashews, and pistachios. Enjoy the delicious taste without overeating by choosing single-portion packets or limiting yourself to a small handful.
- Fruits: the possibilities are endless! Try an apple, peach, pear, strawberries, blueberries, melons, or grapefruit for flavor and nutrients.
- Yogurt and cottage cheese are excellent sources of protein.
- Peanut butter & rice cakes make for a tasty and filling option.
- A green salad is a quick and easy snack, loaded with nutrients and low in calories.

Step 3: S - Structured Meals

Create an eating schedule which will also help with meal planning.

Action:

Pick consistent times for breakfast, lunch, dinner & snacks. Eat meals at about the same time every day.

Eating three meals & one or two snacks per day is a good place to start.

How to Implement:

Here is a structure to follow:

From one meal to another there should be a four hour gap

From one meal to a snack three hour gap

From a snack to a meal three hour gap

Sleep- Your goal should be to get more than seven hours of sleep. The recommended amount of sleep for weight loss is 7-9 hours each day.

Step 4: H- Hack your metabolism

Replace healthy eating with other healthy eating options. It's all about variation - varying the healthy foods you're eating by changing the macros - protein, carbs and fats.

Action:

Change things up to keep the body from adapting.

How to implement:

- » A good way to do this is deciding to have one plant based meal a day or take one week away from animal protein and instead eat more beans, lentils, tofu, and such.
- » You can also eat fewer carbs, drink more water, and eat more raw vegetables instead of cooked ones such as salads.

CONCLUSION

Are you ready to lose weight for good and love your body and your life? You can do what you put your mind to, so believe in yourself and use this book to guide you.

If you need more structured guidance, I would like to invite you to the *Lose Weight Without The Wait* course. This will help you achieve your desired results without drastic dieting. You will hear more about it in the up-coming bonus chapter titled, *"Why You Shouldn't Give Up.*

P.U.S.H
4 PILLAR WEIGHT LOSS SYSTEM

P	P - Purge unhealthy foods Eliminate all processed and highly inflammatory foods for 3 weeks.	Foods to eliminate Alcohol - Wheat products - bread/croissants/bread/cookies/cake, etc Fried Foods - burgers, fries, pizza Other junk - chocolate, sweets, ice cream, granola Unhealthy drinks - juice, lattes, fruit smoothies, energy drinks
U	U - Upgrade quality of foods Focus on eating whole and natural foods	Foods to eat - Carbohydrates: sweet potatoes, yams, potatoes, rice, Weetabix, grits, porridge, carrots, beans, peas, lentils, Weetabix Protein: Chicken, Fish & seafood, beef, lamb, eggs Vegetables: broccoli, green beans/french beans, spinach, kale, cabbage, traditional greens, cauliflower, bok choy
S	S - Structured eating Create an eating schedule. Eat meals at about the same time everyday Eat 3 meals & 1 or 2 snacks per day.	Here is a structure to follow. From 1 meal to another there should be a 4 hr gap From 1 meal to a snack 3 hour gap From a snack to a meal 3 hour gap
H	H - Hack your metabolism Change things up to keep the body from adapting.	Changes should be made to how you eat and cycling macros 1 carb per day 2 carbs per day

Why You Shouldn't Give Up

Bonus Chapter

*"Life is so much more beautiful
and complex than a number on a scale."*
(Munster, n.d.)

BONUS CHAPTER
WHY YOU SHOULDN'T GIVE UP

Is it hard for you to get up this time and figure out how you will lose weight? Is it difficult to look at a full-body shot in the mirror? If so, then you are ready to make a change, and all you need is a little push! I am here to give you the push that you need.

Why You Should Keep Going

- » You are beautiful inside and out. Don't let the number on the scale define who you are.
- » You want to go to the dance recitals and graduations coming up because spending time with friends and family is therapeutic.
- » It is not your fault that you can't stop eating doughnuts and sweets. Depression leads to overeating, and overeating leads to depression. It's a vicious cycle that you don't want to continue.

> » Supplements, weight loss surgery, and fat shrinkage services aren't the answers. Once you get fast weight loss results, how will you keep the weight off long term? They are temporary solutions and quick fixes to a complex problem. It's like using a bandaid for a bullet injury; It will not work if you want permanent solutions.

I know you may be feeling bad, but you are not alone. I love my job because I am able to bring hope to women that feel stuck, and frustrated when nothing else has seemed to work. When I began working with clients, they were overwhelmed and exhausted, but these are some of the testimonials I received after they've been through my transformational weight loss program or course.

From Client 100 Pounds Down [45 Kg Down]

Jane,

"I had given up on ever losing weight after I had tried many diets, but nothing seemed to work. My shoe collection consisted of only flats because I could not walk in heels and my sense of style was lacking. I now enjoy shopping! Today, I walked into a store at the mall, and for once, I didn't hear, *"We don't have your size."* I have so much variety in this smaller size; it's unbelievable. I can finally wear heels without my feet swelling. My husband is so happy for me, and our relationship has become amazing. He even bought me a new ring! God bless you, Jane; you have changed my life."

From Client 10 Weeks Later

"Before Jane's coaching program, I felt heavy, uncomfortable in my clothes, lethargic, and unhappy with what I saw in the mirror. Now, all my clothes fit well, and my wedding ring is looser. Jane, you have taught me how to eat clean, in moderation, and enjoy 'sinful' treats even while losing weight. This is such a thorough and comprehensive program, and I would recommend it to anyone serious about their goals.

In the last 10 weeks of my journey, I have made the following progress

1. Cumulative weight loss of 30 pounds [13.6 Kg]

2. Cumulative inches lost =17 (6 inches from hips, 6 from waist and 5 inches bust)

3. I have moved from a size 16 to 10/12

5. On non-scale victories, I am happier, more alert, and focused. I sleep better, no more swollen feet, no backache, and in control of what I eat. I have glowing skin, I'm energetic, and feel healthier.

Thank you, Jane Mukami."

What You Should Do Next

Whether you use this book and apply everything I have taught you, or you would like to work with me personally, I urge you not to give up. This book is your guide to achieving your weight loss goals. However, if you are ready to take action, I invite you to consider the solution that has helped many women lose weight while enjoying carbohydrates, and without drastic dieting or exercise.

Introducing The Lose Weight Without The Wait 6-Week Course

The *Lose Weight Without The Wait* course will help you fully execute and leverage the power of the P.U.S.H. Weight Loss Method and transform your body, from the inside out, in only six weeks. Here is what you can expect:

Course Overview
SHOPPING LIST

A curated list of proteins, carbs, veggies, and healthy snacks. Enjoy these foods individually, or mix and match for foolproof, healthy meals! This list is full of delicious foods that are affordable on virtually any budget and widely available everywhere in the world.

MEAL PLANNING TOOLS

Have trouble planning ahead for healthy meals? Not a problem! I've designed *two weeks'* worth of mix and match meals that will put you on the fast track to losing stubborn fat that you can use over and over again.

SIX WEEKLY LESSONS

When you know better, you do better. Receive weekly power-packed lessons that will break down the science of fat loss and equip you with the knowledge to help you seamlessly change your eating habits and make healthy living sustainable.

PROGRESS TRACKING

What gets measured gets done. Using my progress tracking tool will help you stay on track as you move closer to your weight loss goal.

WEEKLY INSPIRATION

To keep you focused and motivated to work towards your weight loss goal, weekly inspirational messages will help you get over tough times.

BONUSES: You will also receive three bite-sized guides

<u>Eat Out Guide</u> - Eat out like a pro and have a blast socializing without negatively impacting your waistline.

<u>Travel/Vacation Guide</u> - Navigate life on the go, frequent travel, hotel or resort living without anxiety.

<u>Cravings Guide</u> - Master how to deal with pesky cravings while losing weight.

Who This Course Is For:

Can you relate to any of the following?

- » You want to boost your self-confidence, love how you look, no longer stress about being the largest person at social events, hide under baggy, stretchy, dark-colored clothes, and wear body products to make you look smaller.
- » You want to pursue your dreams and better your life, but you lack energy, mental clarity, and excitement for your job.
- » You're unfulfilled, feel helpless, and wonder how or why other women can lose weight and live their best life, but you can't seem to do it.
- » You have low self-esteem or a non-existent social life that makes you feel alone, or your relationship with your partner is falling apart because you lack energy or have zero interest in sexual relations.

What's Your Goal?

Whatever your "why" is for losing weight, remember to let your why be larger than the number on the scale. The decision is up to you.

Here are a few lifestyle results, Non-Scale Victories (NSVs) others have received who once felt lost, just like you.

Testimonial
Confidence, Clarity & Optimism

"I used to feel fat, not sleeping well, bloated, and tired. Now I feel amazing and confident like I could conquer the world! Jane is very knowledgeable, and she has taught me that weight loss, first of all, is a science. It all begins in the mind, and if you conquer your mindset, there is nothing you can't do! Her guidance has been priceless."

Energetic, Happy & Confidence

"I used to have low energy, knee pain, and couldn't sleep well at night. After losing 41 pounds, [19 kilos] and now fitting clothes from six years ago, size 8 from a size 18, I feel happy and confident. Jane has helped me understand nutrition and how the body works. Her program has been the best investment ever and has made this an amazing year."

Happy, Healthy & Grateful

"I had labs done yesterday, and prolactin levels are now 30.9 when weighing 146.5 pounds. Before the program two months ago, I was 167 pounds, and my prolactin levels were 88. The doctor is extremely happy with my progress and told me to keep doing what I've been doing. Thank you so much Jane! Your program has restored my health, and I remain forever grateful."

If you are READY to leap, then scan the QR code below or visiting the link to learn more about the *LOSE WEIGHT WITHOUT THE WAIT* Course

https://www.loseweightwithoutthewait.com/6-week-course

A Note From The Author Jane Mukami

Thank you for purchasing this book. Whether you follow this book and use it to lose weight or you join my 6-week course, remember to keep going and never give up.

I am passionate about helping women lose weight to look good and feel great. They can increase self-confidence and self-love and live a happy and exciting life.

I am a multi-award-winning health coach, author, speaker, and creator of **The P.U.S.H. Weight Loss Method.** I am fully committed to my purpose of coaching women through weight loss and body transformation for life transformation. Please keep in touch and follow me for tips.

XO, Jane

https://instagram.com/fitkenyangirl

Author's Bio

Jane Mukami is a passionate and multi-award-winning health coach, and author. Born in Nairobi, Kenya, she decided to remain in Atlanta, Georgia, over two decades ago after completing her college education. After losing weight, Jane became determined to share the life-altering power of healthy living with others.

Jane exhibits an infectious enthusiasm for her cause and is adamant that health should be a priority at any age – even after 60! She was recently recognized as one of *Okay Africa's Top 100 African Women*. She has won numerous awards, including the Health & Fitness Award 2019 ACHI Awards, Health Influencer Award 2019, Journey Awards also in 2019, and the Health & Fitness Coach Award from Africa Women's Leader Awards in 2018.

Jane is passionate about changing the narrative of aging and motivating people to live healthier lives as she continues her mission to impact 1 million women worldwide.

REFERENCES

Frankel, B. (n.d.). *- your diet is a bank account. good food... -* . BrainyQuote. https://www.brainyquote.com/quotes/bethenny_frankel_482602

Hippocrates. (2023, July 8). *Statustown.* https://statustown.com/englishstatus/6532/

Horace. (n.d.). *Good health ideas.* Pacefood group. https://pacefoodgroup.com/good-healthy-ideas/

Hyman, M. M. (2019, November 13). *Why don't they teach nutrition in medical school?* Dr. Mark Hyman. https://drhyman.com/blog/2018/09/07/why-dont-they-teach-nutrition-in-medical-school/

Jaret, P. (2014, March 31). *The arthritis diet: How excess weight damages your joints.* WebMD. https://www.webmd.com/arthritis/features/weight-joint-pain#:~:text=Excess%20weight%20puts%20added%20stress,rheumatology%20at%20Johns%20Hopkins%20University

Mark Hyman, M. (2019, December 5). *You can't exercise your way out of a bad diet, but here are 7 reasons why exercise is still important.* Dr. Mark Hyman. https://drhyman.com/blog/2015/09/11/you-cant-exercise-your-way-out-of-a-bad-diet-but-here-are-7-reasons-why-exercise-is-still-important/

Motivation Power. (2016, March 2). *The distance between who I am and who I want to be is separated...* Daily Inspirational Quotes.

https://www.dailyinspirationalquotes.in/2014/02/the-distance-between-who-i-am-and-who-i-want-to-be-is-separated-only-by-my-actions-and-words-anonymous-inspiring-quotes/

Munster, T. (n.d.). *10 quotes about body positivity*. The Best of Life. https://bestoflife.com/quotes-about-body-positivity/

Pollan, M. (n.d.). *Food is not just fuel*. AZ Quotes. https://www.azquotes.com/quote/797681

Robert J. Reier, D. (2018, July 23). *"every time you eat or drink, you are either feeding disease or fighting it."* Healthy Harford. https://www.healthyharford.org/beware-diet-is-a-four-letter-word-2

Shomon, M. (2023, August 1). How less sleep affects your metabolism and prevents weight loss. Verywell Health. https://www.verywellhealth.com/sleep-more-lose-weight-3233044

Stevens, C. C. (n.d.). *A quote from the lies about truth*. Goodreads. https://www.goodreads.com/quotes/7304033-if-nothing-changes-nothing-changes-if-you-keep-doing-what

Taylor Lippman [taylorlippman]. (2021, October, 2021). Defined as - "A mental illness involving obsessive focus on a perceived flaw in appearance." [Photograph]. Instagram. https://www.instagram.com/p/CUvnTnCptbL/

Totie Fields. (n.d.). BrainyQuote. https://www.brainyquote.com/authors/totie-fields-quotes

Made in the USA
Columbia, SC
27 September 2023